CW00455966

Magical Thoughts and Reflections

Magical Thoughts and Reflections

An Illustrated Poetry Anthology

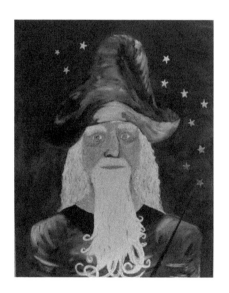

Karen Old

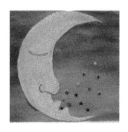

Copyright © 2023 by Karen Old

All rights reserved.
No part of this book may be reproduced or used in
any manner without written permission of the copyright
owner except for the use of quotations in a book review.

For more information, contact: healingartinfo@yahoo.com

First paperback edition 2023

Book cover design by Publishing Push
Edited by Steve Hall and Celia Speirs
Illustrated by Karen Old

978-1-80541-115-4 (paperback)
978-1-80541-117-8 (hardback)
978-1-80541-116-1 (ebook)

Contents

Foreword

Magical Thoughts and Reflections is a thought-provoking and empowering collection of poems. The way in which it has been written feels caring and personal and comes from the author's spiritual heart. The book is clearly written and channelled with spirit to help with healing. It is an aid to removing negative thought patterns in order to promote clear thinking.

Maybe we shouldn't have favourites, but I did. There were two in particular I couldn't get out of my mind. 'Having a Laugh' was unexpected and made me giggle, while 'The Rush' I liked for its simplicity. That's not to take away from the fact that each poem has a message and a teaching.

The illustrations and photos add to the authenticity and pure message of the poetry. I love the way in which the poems have been written with gentle humour. The hidden or not so hidden messages stayed in my mind for hours, or even days.

Sometimes I laughed out loud; other times my soul was touched and a tear came to my eye. Without doubt, it's a book to read and one that will stay on my shelf to be read over and over.

A uniquely powerful book.

Nicola Hall

Psychic Medium

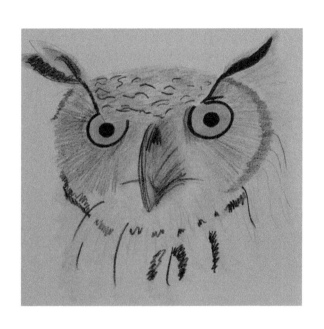

Acknowledgments

There are many people to thank for the final publication of this book. From the outset Bev, Deb, Mary and Sam were more than determined to see writing commence. During the early review Ady, Alison, Kieran and Nicola were encouraging, supportive and constructively critical. Steve has been meticulously studious with his editorial skill and endlessly patient with his attention and advice. Celia has worked like a hawk to iron out editorial issues. George and Annie have given generously of their time to read and record. Ivee from Publishing Push has worked with the Publishing Push Team to co-ordinate this project in a professional, friendly manner. Indeed with unfailing courtesy and forbearance.

I would like to thank all of you so very much for without you *'Magical Thoughts and Reflections'* just would not have happened.

Preface

Psychic Medium 1 - You need to be writing!

Self - Really?

Psychic Medium 2 - I am being urged to tell you to write!

Self - Thank you.

Psychic Medium 3 - Have you ever thought of writing?

Self – No, not really.

Psychic Medium 4 - You are going to be writing short pieces. Like blogs.

Self – Oh, that it is interesting.

Psychic Medium 5 - You are going to write a book!

Self – Sorry, I can't quite see it.

Psychic Medium 6 - I am going to be buying your book?

Self - Not sure about that.

Psychic Medium 7 - I can see you with a long feather. A quill. I feel you are going to write.

Self - I have been told this.

Psychic Medium 8 - You are going to write.

Self - I don't really want to write. I have enough to do.

Psychic Medium 9 - 'They' want you to write.

Self - Would you mind asking 'them' what it is they want me to write about?

Psychic Medium 10 - You are going to write a book. It is not a normal book. It is very different.

Self - I keep being told this, but I don't know what it is they want me to write or indeed how to start.

Psychic Medium 10 - Just get a sheet of paper and a pen, sit quiet and write.

Self - Easy!

Introduction

When you are a spiritual person, you work, rest and play alongside other spiritual people. Over the past few years, I have had these conversations and many more in a similar vein.

Magical Thoughts and Reflections is the result of sitting in the quiet with paper and pen. What came was inspiration to produce a poetry collection of different styles. Styles ranging from the limerick and Japanese haiku to free verse and rhyming with different patterns. Each poem is the vector of a lesson or a message about personal growth or professional development. Each piece is accompanied by artwork that complements the subject in some way. Some of the artwork, particularly the portraits, were also produced by sitting in the quiet and waiting for inspiration. This could be described, by some, as channelling. Some of the poems are powerful in their emotional stimulus. Some will make you laugh, and some will make you cry. All of them will stimulate contemplation.

Happy Reading!

Words From Spirit

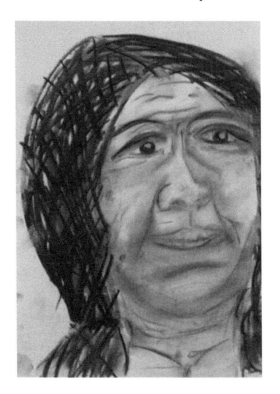

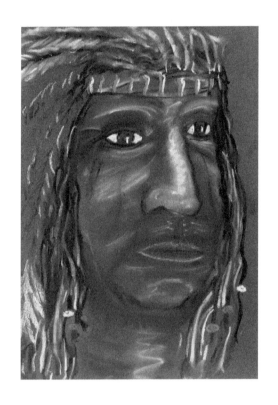

Thought for the day!
Fly High

Fly as high as the eagle.
Walk with the ground beneath bare feet.
Swim with the fish and the mammal.
Love and cherish the earth.
Tomorrow is another day, for now.

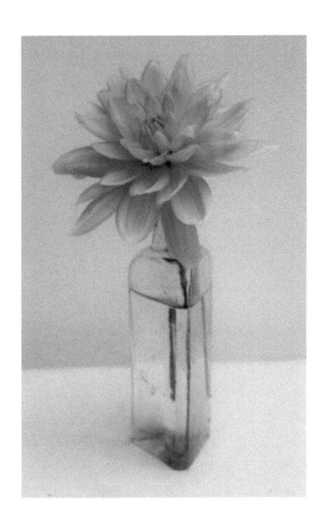

Grass Roots - Simplicity

The iron is a weight to remove the creases from the cloth.
The chandelier lights the home of the decadent.
Skin and bone are the trappings of mere mortals.
The skin does not see the crease.
The bone does not see the crystal.
Frills are an added encumbrance to peace.
Simplicity is the way.

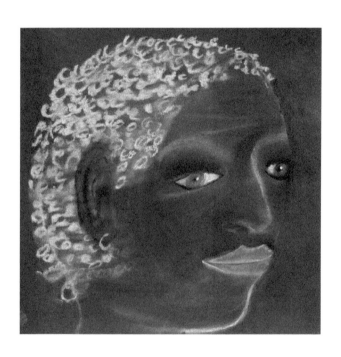

Hullabaloo

Time! Time! Time! Time!
Hullabaloo, Hullabaloo, Hullabaloo!
Time! Time! Time! Time!
Hullabaloo! Stop!
Wait awhile with me,
And listen,
Really listen.
What does your soul say today?

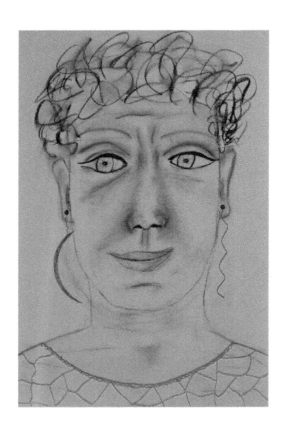

Authentic

Who are we to deny our true selves?
Who are we to cover our light?
Who are we to live by another's ideal?
Who are we?
Strive to dance to your own tune.
Express your truth no matter.
Stand up and be seen in your full glory.
Be proud to be individual!
Be proud to be different!
Be proud to be authentic!
Be modest, be kind, but above all be true!

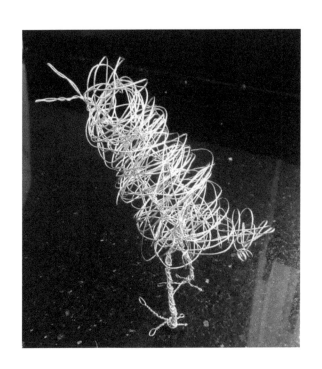

The Rush

The early bird catches the worm,
But the late bird watches the entertainment.

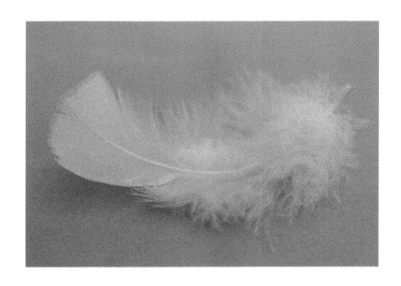

The Soul

It is only when the soul speaks,
We understand who we truly are.

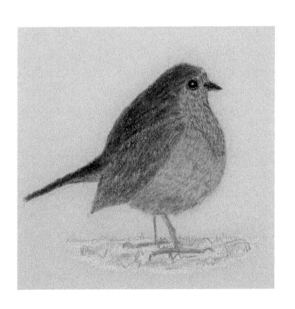

Seek

Seek the quiet
Seek the still.
Seek the pure,
Seek the modest.
Seek the meek.
They hold the key to the truth.
Truth is love.

Being Human

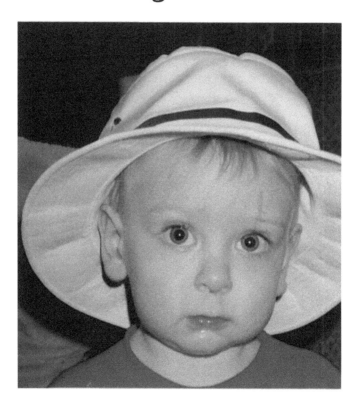

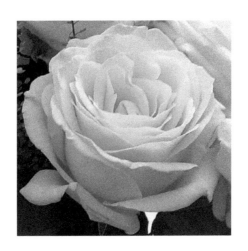

Life's Sensation

Taking a breath,
The journey begins.
In a wash of love,
Wrapped in cloth.
We have no sins, no ire, no wrath.

Walking the path,
So straight and narrow,
With highs and lows like ridge and furrow,
Creates the marks in brows
And foreheads. Torment.

But oh! What wondrous joys there are
If only we can see beyond our noses.
The birds, the sky, the roses!
And smell the freesia or the pansy –
Then life could be quite dandy.

Or taste the orange and the lime –
Then life will be just fine.
Hearing notes upon the breeze
Of the fingers on the keys
Of ebony and ivory.

Power of the human touch
Is something that we clutch.
To feel the skin on skin,
Is something akin to elation.
Sense sensation, the foundation of our being.

Our reason for seeing, hearing, smelling,
For tasting and, above all, for holding, for hugging.
For loving.
And when the last breath is taken
At the end of our life's track
'Twill be good to know our senses
Were put to good use, looking back.

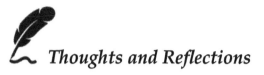 *Thoughts and Reflections*

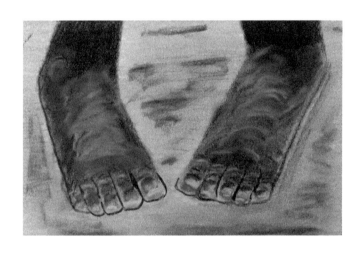

Haiku

Rockets blast moonwards.
The girl walks shoeless in heat
To fetch the water.

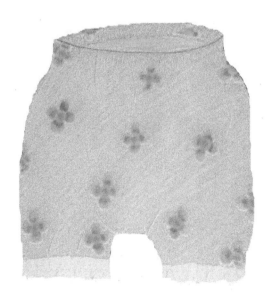

Having a Laugh

There was a young lady called Lunar
Whose stitching undid in her bloomer.
She felt oh so silly
And remarkably chilly
As she bent down revealing a mooner.

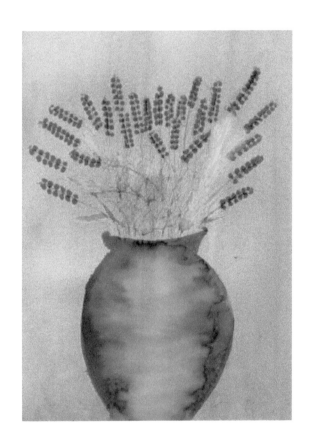

Mind Games

Sometimes it's hard to stop the slip
Of the smile that's fixed upon the lip.
We place it there for all to see
That we are happy.

We place it there to charm, beguile,
That dazzling, gleaming, sparkling smile.
The muscles in our jaws do ache,
But we are happy!

Our eyes reveal the inner state,
The cumbersome turmoil of life's weight.
It reaches out through iris blue,
Disclosing the discomfort.

It is hard to retain in place,
That smile that curves upon the face.
The brain can have a different view,
That all's not well.

What is the purpose of this façade
When life, at times, can be so hard?
Protection, reassurance, delusion maybe;
All is not how we want it.

The mind is but an untamed beast
That struts about the place unleashed.
We catch it, then put on the collar
To bring it to order.

The tools we use to train the brain
Can make you feel whole again.
Laughing yoga, CBT, absolute positivity
Can refresh the aching mind.

It is not easy! We have to fight
To gain control with all our might.
But persevere. Success will come.
You will feel genuinely happy!

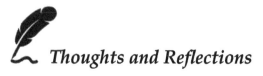 *Thoughts and Reflections*

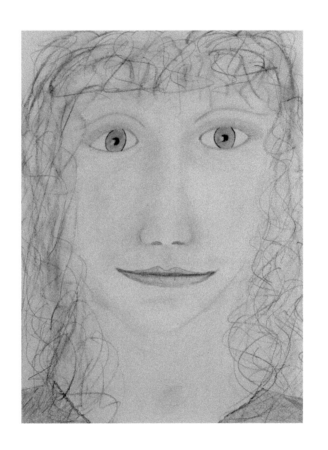

Square Peg

Everyone is talking,
Competing
Speaking
Drivelling.

I can't find my way
Through the conversing.
I'm tensing.
Sensing.

Regretting
Coming to this meeting.
I'm heating,
Stewing.

Flustered.
Can't get words out.
Can't spout.
Dumbfounded.

Confounded.
Where do I begin?
Don't fit in.
Head splitting.

Mind racing.
I am different.
Rejection,
Alienation.

Isolation –
There it is.
What a swizz!
How did I get in?

Camouflaged,
No guard,
Through the door,
Unsuspecting.

Rearranging thought patterns,
Must admit
Defeat.
Retreat.

Impeach.
Must play fair.
Find the hole that's square!
Accepting,
Engulfing,
Embracing.
At peace, like with like.
Mending. Sighing. Relaxing.

Thoughts and Reflections

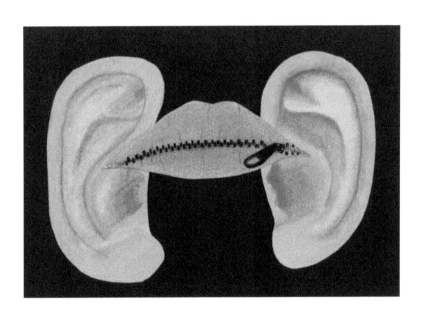

Two Ears. One Mouth

Talking less and listening more enables one to comprehend what is being said.
To comprehend is to understand what is going on in someone's head.
To understand means we can act, if need be, to help another.
In this society, the selfless are few and far between.
Too often people want to talk, they don't want to listen.
Listening takes attention from the self.
For many, the self is the most important.
When the quiet man talks, be ready to embrace what is being said.
Be ready to listen.
Avoid the man who talks incessantly. They will not miss you.
The loudest vessel is the emptiest.
Avoid the men who talk loudly to compete. To gain status.
Be thankful in the knowledge there is no room for you.

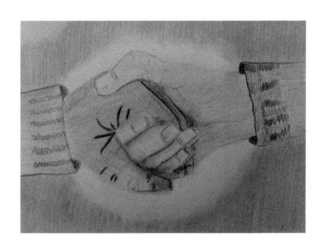

The Error of our Ways

Serious error, blunder,
Turns the stomach wall.
Heart begins to race and thump,
Skin begins to crawl.
Nausea rises as implications dawn,
Emotions in turmoil,
Nervous system torn.

Regret, repent, admonishment,
Will not reset the clock.
Time is gone, deed is done.
You are reeling from the shock.

Shackle of guilt is heavy,
Weighing down on both your feet.
Makes normal life impossible,
Your tendency to retreat.

Devastation is so black and hopeless,
Reproach, disgrace, unhelpful.
There is a desperate need to find
Something more insightful.

Find the gleam of golden thread,
It runs right through the gloom.
It will lead you to the very key
To unlock you from the tomb.

In life we are always learning.
From the dark depths find the lesson.
Cocoon yourself in tutorage.
Find a way to give expression
To your thoughts and fears and phobias
That dangle in your mind.
You will emerge more learned,
And more able, you will find.
To approach a problem differently,
You will take a different view.
The Error will become your friend
And will walk alongside you.

To remind you we are human,
And to err is what may be,
Inside all of us, at some time,
Straight lines become shaky.

Be kindly to another one
Who has made a big mistake.
Wrap them carefully up in love
To reduce their own heartache.

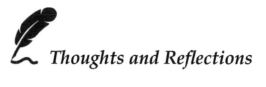

Thoughts and Reflections

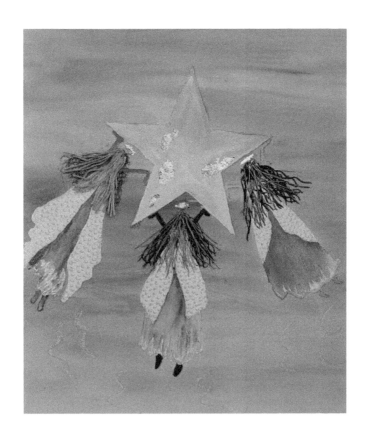

Sharing

Altogether cast the net.
Haul in the load.
We achieve much more in unison.
Submit to your fellow man.
Avoid fiercely guarding your own project for personal
prestige.
Generously share the burden of hard work.
Others can gain a sense of satisfaction that they have
helped.
Others can be reassured that they are needed.
Others can develop their own skills and knowledge.
The man who seeks all the adoration for himself misses out
on teamwork and camaraderie.
Give your children tasks.
They need them as part of their development.
They will gain a greater understanding of what is involved
and a greater appreciation for you.
Celebrating achievement in a group is much more fun!

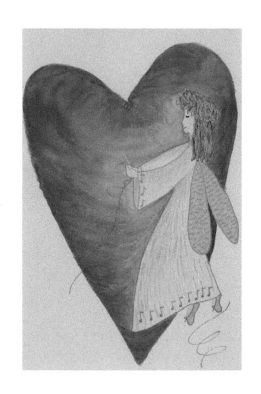

Coping

Here comes the sun. It's not always cast out.
It hides behind black clouds in moments of doubt.
It is there though its brightness cannot be seen,
To reveal itself gently when the skies become clean.
There are times in our lives when we worry and grieve,
For our nearest and dearest and the path that they lead.

We'll tussle and turn, churning over in mind
What action to take to keep them aligned
With the goals that we have, with the values we trust.
But sometimes the back seat is the place that we must
Reside in, to observe the events that reveal,
Requiring us to have strong nerves of steel.

We are not the drivers of another's path.
We advise and support through the aftermath.
It is not for us to worry about the way that they tread.
The energy can be put to better use instead.
Reversing your thoughts to allow things to be
Removes, at a stroke, your anxiety.

Instead, reassure your floundering mind
To take a step back is hardly unkind.
Recognise that the sun will continue to shine

In moments of grief, with help from Divine.
Resources to cope will arrive at your gate,
To help you sit up, to keep your back straight.

To see what's required, to pull you together,
To make you much stronger from this point, forever.

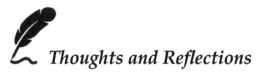 *Thoughts and Reflections*

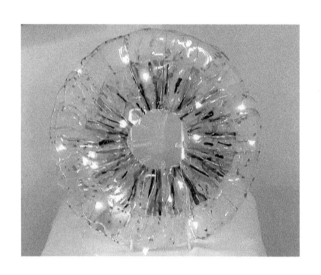

The Human Gaze

Born with silver spoon,
Walk with head held high.
Avoid the glance of others,
With momentum passing by.

Homeless in the gutter,
Nursing head down low.
Avoid the glance of others,
Who are moving to and fro.

Lack of eye contact in the former
Is wrapped in selfish guilt.
While the latter avoids the gaze,
Humiliating pain up to the hilt.

What must it take
To stretch the focus and look upon another?
Gaze into the coloured iris
Of a troubled human brother.

For here resides the soul,
Naked in all its glory.
It tells of all the anguish,
Pain and the whole life story.

Troubles traverse a race,
A creed, a class, a population.
Comfort comes from reaching out,
Regardless of our station.

Success, to bridge the gap,
Is to find the living key.
To reach the man beneath the skin,
You must open your eyes and see!

Family

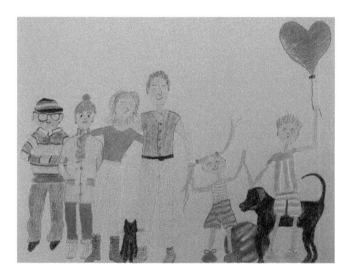

The family – Clothed in love. The fabric of our being.

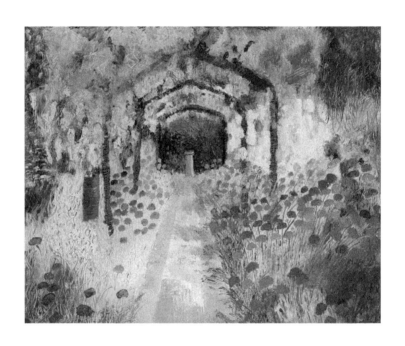

Garden of Love

Planting a garden is done for a life.
Much like a marriage when a man takes a wife.
Here come the bulbs in the first light of spring.
Sap running high as he places the ring.
Bluebells and crocus colour the way,
Radiating joy as they live day to day.
Shoots converge quickly with the sun at its peak.
Children will follow. Lives full of mystique.
They follow their path through the smooth and the rough,
Like ivy that curves round the trunk stiff and tough.
The fabric of family makes a strong tether,
As roots in the soil hold on in bad weather.
The autumn winds blow. The fruit hits the ground.
Children leave home. The house carries no sound.
There is grief, there is mourning, as the house becomes bare.
The trappings of childhood are no longer there.
But just like the leaves that replenish the Earth,
The quiet time leads to a tranquil rebirth.
There is space to prune hard to make the bough stronger.
Interests develop. There is sadness no longer.
Winter's frost on the ground magically twinkles,
While the love in our hearts sparkles through wrinkles.
The man that I cherish gardens with care,
And the love that we've nurtured will always grow there.

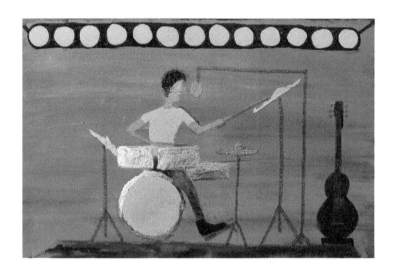

Gratitude

From a distance, I can say these things to you,
My lovely boy.
Life is not a trifle to be played with,
Like a toy.

It has its grave, grave elements
That throw up disarray,
That make it difficult to function,
To get right through the day.

It's therefore most important
To stop and see the light
That shines upon you unbeknown,
Through the day and through the night.

You have two eyes to see the path
To let you safely tread.
You have two ears to hear the sound
That earns your daily bread.

You have the voice to speak, to sing,
To give your point of view.
You have a home, you have a job,
Some would envy you.

Your muscles move your bony mass
To let you walk and run.
Your taste buds can be tickled,
Placing food upon your tongue.

Your nose can scent the flowers,
The pizza and perfume.
Your smile is so radiant,
It can light the darkest room.

But most importantly you have
The love of family and friends.
It's time to cast off negative thoughts
And with yourself make amends.

Be grateful for God-given gifts,
Celebrate them every day.
Being positive is not always easy,
But essentially, it's 'the way'.

And when those murky thoughts appear,
Go catch them with a net!
Replace them with something wonderful,
A joyous, new mindset!

Before you drop this in the bin,
I have but one request.
To sit and reassure yourself
Sometimes mothers do know best.

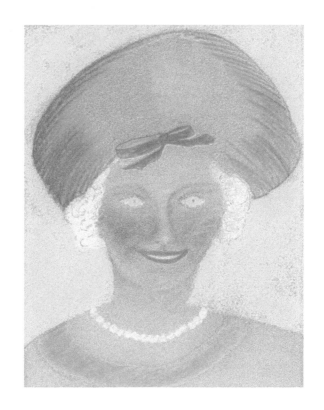

'What's meant for you won't go by you!'

'What's meant for you won't go by you,'
My Grandma used to say
As she gently stroked my hair
And brushed my tears away.
It's something that has stayed with me
And stood the test of time.
I find I use it gently,
When required from time to time.

Don't fret my little one!
It did not go your way.
What will come to you tomorrow
Is not meant for you today.
There is no point in crying
Or steaming through your ears.
It's best to find the error.
Look beyond how it appears.
To fail is the reason
We can learn an awful lot,
To develop into adulthood
From the safely swinging cot.
You'll emerge a little wiser,
More attuned to what's required,
With improvement on the Western Front

From a brain that's been rewired.
Although it looks bleak in the present,
There is something very true:
With Destiny at play,
What's meant will not pass you.

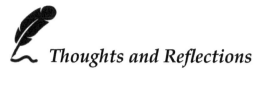 *Thoughts and Reflections*

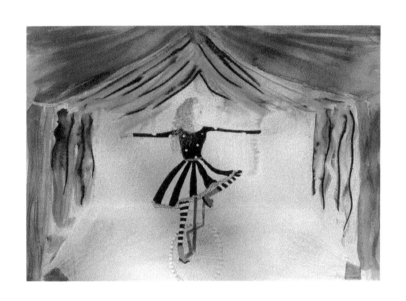

The Actress

'I can't do this,' the actress said,
Sporting tear-stained face.
'The odds are stacked against me,
My scripts are in disgrace.
I don't know where to start to climb
This shaky, flimsy ladder,
And when I start to think of it,
It simply makes me madder!

My ruminating brain has me
Spinning round and round.
It gives me such a headache
Which thumps and grinds and pounds.
'Find an agent,' someone says,
'Cos it's just like riding a bike.'
Well, it shows how little they know –
It's like a hundred-mile hike!

The monologues they take me
From *Macbeth* to *A Doll's House*.
But how I characterise these pieces,
Be it lion or church mouse,
Has me going round in circles,
Different shades of purple hues.

Monkey brain is jumping hurdles,
And I'm feeling quite confused.

It's not the thought of being
Another blazing star.
But to use God's given talents
To be authentically who you are.
I am a comedic actress.
Singer. Dancer. Yes, it's true.
And I wish to use my talents
To stand tall in front of you.

So, I need to sort my head out,
Worry less and overcome.
The fear I have of failure
Makes me feel I want to run.
I can achieve some freedom
From this pacing animal enclosure.
Strict time-bound plans and targets
Will lead to more positive exposure.
And so, what if I don't succeed?
Have I got to run and hide?
No! I can safely reassure myself,
In the knowledge that I've tried!'

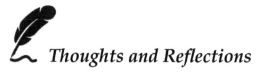 *Thoughts and Reflections*

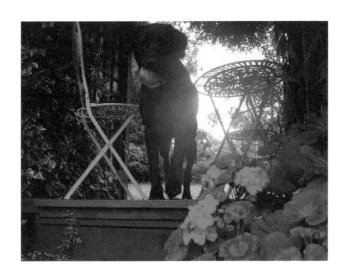

Alf

You wouldn't take a bull into a china shop,
Yet we bought him into our home.
A tonne of skin, muscle, bone.
A large, vital, natural force,
Resembling something of a Great Dane or small horse.
His fur was black but his eyes so bright
You could see him walking in the dark at night.
And his teeth so white against his tongue,
A beautiful pink, like bubble gum.
When still, his ears lay softly on his face,
Pulling back in the wind when he gave chase.
And boy he could run! Outrun them all!
To get his stick or grab his ball.
Returning, though, was not his wish,
He'd roll in fox poo or eat old fish.
Or run in circles round the lake,
Giggling quietly at his 'mickey take'.
We'd call him frantically, you know,
And every so often his head would show.
It would bob up through the rambling grass.
At our expense he'd have such a laugh!
Getting home was no mean feat:
He'd decline the cheese, the sausage, the meat.
He'd decline all treats to be truly free.

There was no free spirit such as he.
And here we stand without him now.
His ashes are his last one bow.
But there are remnants of his being,
If you take the time for really seeing.
There are tooth prints in the furniture and scratches on the wall,
Several balls in the garden and dog hair in the hall.
And there they'll stay so we fondly remember,
Our loving dog Alfie from this day, forever.

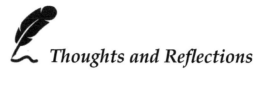 *Thoughts and Reflections*

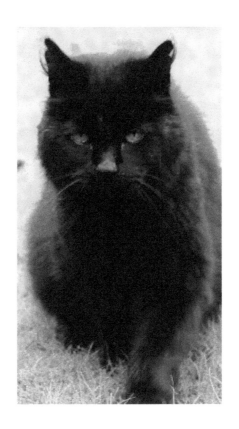

Minky

Black cat, green eyes,
Sits in the garden and quickly spies
A rustle and a silver back
Of a mouse scurrying along its track.
But write its will, if human would,
And make it watertight it should!
For that black cat is a mean machine.
He'll use that mouse for his cuisine.
But there's a part that makes him shiver.
He'll spit out the stomach and the liver.
But do not fear they'll go to waste.
The cat will move with lightning haste
To place them on our front door mat!
That generous, green-eyed, black-furred cat.

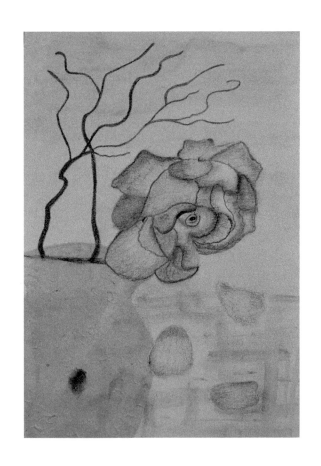

Acceptance

Accept your loved one lies in wait.
By St. Peter, they straddle the gate.
Accept one foot feels the air,
The other in ether unaware.
Dementia like a wilted flower,
Petals fall with loss of power.
Cause the eyes to see in double.
Monkeys, rhino! All sorts of trouble.
Accept they lose the words to say.
But love you? They do every day.

Balance moves across the portal,
When the soul departs from this mere mortal.
Accept they'll pass, for die they must.
We all will turn to ash and dust.
Accept they'll join the spirit world,
New ways of being soon unfurled.
Accepting lets you free your mind.
Stress and guilt get left behind.
Accept you'll meet another day,
When you yourself will walk this way.

Friendship

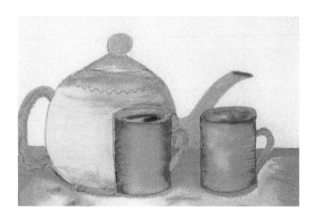

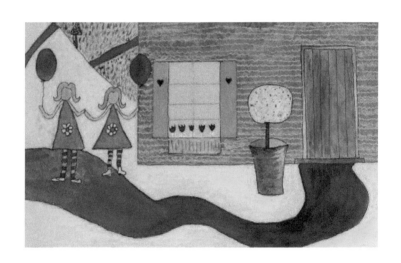

What is a friend?

What is a friend?
Someone who will draw near when the going gets tough.
Someone who buoys you up when the going gets rough.
Someone who is there at four in the morning.
Someone who listens, suppressing the yawning.
Someone who gives without expecting back.
Someone who sticks with you steadfast through the flack.
Someone who looks to encourage and nurture.
Someone who will be there sometime in the future.
Someone who gives a kind, honest word.
Someone whose intentions are clearly unblurred.
Someone whose friendship you would be proud of.
Someone who gives unconditional love.
Could you be the 'someone' that you are looking for?
Could you be the friend that someone longs for?

Work

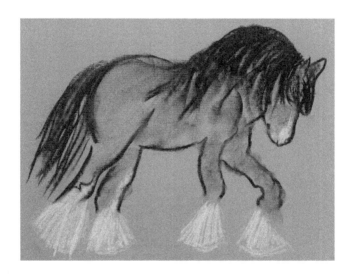

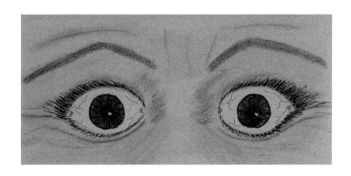

The Line Manager

I've observed in some line managers,
They have some things in common.
They are working their way to the top,
From the depths of scaley bottom.

They'll draw you in on your first day,
And flatter to deceive.
Introduce you as the 'wondrous one'.
They think you're so naïve.

They'll trample on all heads and toes
To get to number one.
To them it's just a blood sport,
Packed with tremendous fun!

Engrossed in their SMART targets,
They will shut themselves away,
Analysing facts and figures:
'Do projected match today's?'

And if successful,
They will stop and think a while,
Congratulate themselves. It is
Due to their management style.

But if these figures should fall short,
Prepare to buckle up.
They are planning how to crack the whip,
While sipping coffee from their cup.

They will hound you in the morning,
They will hound you after dark.
You will wear the badge of stress
Like branded cattle wear the mark.

For the blame for shortfall figures
Will be laid firmly at your door.
Your conscientious ethic
Counts for nothing anymore.

They see you as a challenge
And set about their mission
To wear you down into the ground
While elevating their position.

Over-inflated predicted figures
They pointedly refuse to see.
'Ambition is so important,'
They acknowledge. 'Look at me!'

It takes a lot of bravery
To walk away from that,
To look them in the eye
And say, 'Stick it up your hat.'

But sometimes it is necessary
To genuinely take heed.
To walk out, head held high, with dignity,
Is probably what you need.

Energy Medicine

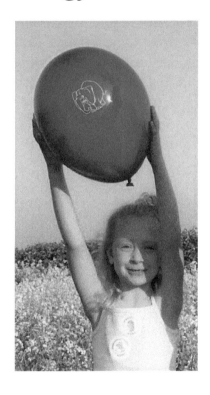

A section for the holistic therapist or for those who have an interest in all types of complementary therapy. 'Humans have a vital force that animates the body.' This is one of the key beliefs. The vital force can be stimulated by a variety of things, including vibrations of different frequencies and thought patterns.

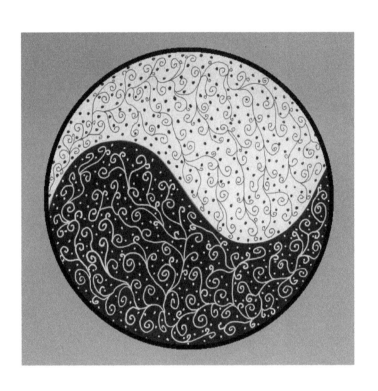

Fight the Good Fight

Out of chaos the teardrops stood,
Faced each other to discuss who was good.
Yin replied, 'It's me, you see.
I am far more passive than you can be!
My colour is black. I like the shade.
I love it when the moon's displayed!
My energy low, I am cool and still.
I can gauge when to fall and retreat at will.
When tragedy calls, I know how to hide.
You'll find me quiet on the Northern side.
My energy female, yielding and gentle.
A mother's love, softly sentimental.'

Yang looked on and shook his head.
'It's not as simple as that!' he said.
'For I am light and strong and bright,
And I can push with all my might.
Ascent, advance and climbing high
To touch the sun, so warm and dry,
Are things that I would like to do,
For I am far more challenging than you!
Comedic elements are quite clear.
You'll never find me at the rear
But out in front I will be seen.
I feel my energy reigns supreme.'

The two embraced and tossed and tussled.
They flew right up and became quite puzzled
Because as they formed a flying ball,
They ascended, up, then began to fall.
They pondered on their friendly spat;
They needed each other and that was that.
For though they are an opposite force,
They combine as one in intercourse.
As day follows night and night follows day,
Order comes from disarray.
As stillness comes from a period of riot,
Parties are followed by peace and quiet.
As the pair's relationship begins to mend,
They recognise each other as close friends.
They interlink in unity,
To form the symbol of Tai Chi.

Thoughts and Reflections

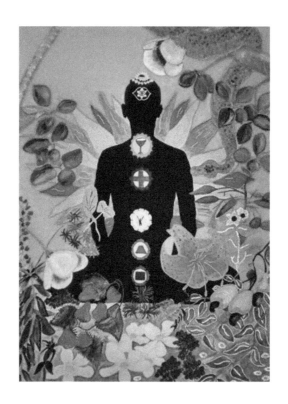

The Healer

She crawls upon her belly,
The essence of snake.
Avoiding staring eyes
Of those that might make
Light of her candour,
Ridicule her trust.
Doubting herself
Is something she must
Avoid at all costs.
Nurturing fervour,
Her craft is her passion.
Reactions unnerve her.
Strive as she does
To help the sick,
The fierce damning insults
Cut to the quick.
Sometime in the future,
People may see
There is good in this medicine,
For you and for me.
Until such a time
She'll continue to slide
Between a rock and a hard place
While her hands are well tied.

The establishment continues
To dish out the pills,
Which are not always the solution
To disease, woes and ills.
Sometimes we just need
To take a different view,
To apply an essence
Of a unique hue.
And what of that person
Who has no relief?
Who flounders with
Sceptical, staunch disbelief
In something that
Might just save the day,
Causing that symptom
To pass straight away?
That person continues
Along their own track.
But others more desperate
Might turn the clock back
And seek out some help
From unlikely places.
Perhaps the snake will rise
And look in the faces
Of those who have rubbished
Her kind existence.

Of those who have
Demonstrated pure resistance
To a shade so precise
To make healing its goal,
To a colour so gentle
It touches the soul.

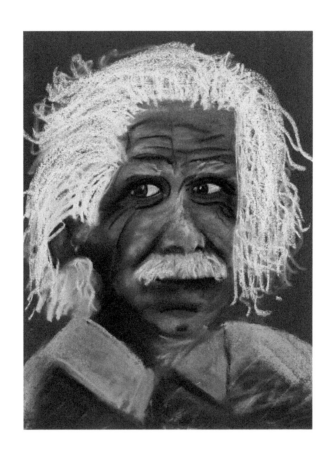

E=mc2

E=mc^2 so Einstein said,
A multitude of figures
Swimming round inside his head.
The fact is all of matter
Has an energetic base
That comes to Earth
From somewhere in the depths of outer space.

He determined that the Constant
Was the super speed of light,
That comes to Earth from the sun,
And when squared, it makes it right.
The number for the speed of light
Is far from being small:
At 300,000km per second squared,
It's huge! So all in all,
It therefore means a tiny mass
Can store a massive lot
Of energy in Joules
To be released in aliquots.

For energy destruction is not a possible task.
How can we harness power?
Is something we should ask.

Trituration and succession give the energy route out
To vibrate within the sitter,
Casting out all doubt.
The secret is the resonance
Of waves that synchronise
And sway with amplitude increased
As symptoms minimise.

Healing is so critical:
Energy moves right to the core.
The disturbance is cast out,
And you are better than before.
Our ability to use this course
Is constantly criticised
By those whose minds are narrowed.
This technique they publicly despise.

If only they could see a way
To work for greater good,
Researching the hypothesis
Scientifically – as they should!
Humans would be better placed
To use the tools in hand.
Convention and alternative,
They'd have both at their command.

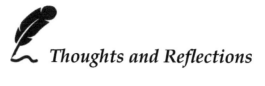 *Thoughts and Reflections*

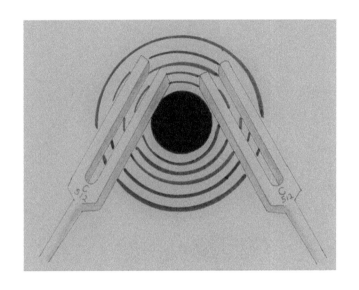

Like attracts like!

Glum, downtrodden, top of the heap!
Licking wounds. Out. Downbeat.
No way out. Catastrophic!
All is dark, bleak, demonic.
Sending out the wish to change,
A life that needs a rearrange.
But, just like tuning forks vibrate,
Attracting another at the same rate,
And as those waves do meet in phase,
The amplitude is slowly raised.
The state of *Bleak House* soldiers on,
Even though you wish it gone.

Instead, you need to turn the tide
And change your thoughts from deep inside.
Plant the seeds of what you want.
Focus hard without guilt or prompt.
Feel it, touch it. See it's truth.
Imagine it right with you. Not aloof.
Feel the joy and satisfaction it brings
To make those tuning forks start to ring.
The resonance darts out to universal force,
Returning ten-fold to put you on course
For a life that's filled with awe and wonder.
The dark times can be put asunder.

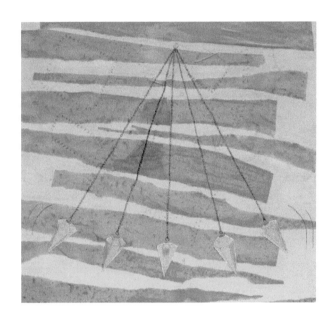

Polarity Pendulum

Elemental human state,
Within, the vital force vibrates.
Swinging back and forth with ease,
In health. Impeded, brings dis-ease.

The pendulum's freedom doth get stuck,
To leave you feeling, 'What bad luck!'
It oscillates between a polar pair.
Extremes uppermost. Balance rare.

Observe the hard and rigid Earth
Exemplified by gut and girth.
Its role is to discriminate,
Digest, solidify and defecate.

At times you feel things move so slow
And wish a hardened wedge would flow.
Flow it will, expanding fast.
Dissolving lines, the wedge will pass.

With Water's frank and forceful tide,
Filtering, accepting, no place to hide.
It flows to every nook and crack,
Upends the root, the hoof, the shack.

Emotionally, it's plain to see,
Chinks form in steel armoury.
Stiff upper lips crumble and melt,
Salt tears pour forth with emotion felt.

Fire can rage in another's head,
Bringing passion and love or anger instead.
Igniting beckons laughter, rejoicing,
Ecstasy, passion or wrath in voicing.

Fire state falls into depths of despair,
Love unrequited will lead one to Air.
The brain is divorced from cool, cold reason.
This is darkness and bleakness, the winter season.

Lungs suffocate as grief takes its strong hold,
Claustrophobia threatens. There's a need to be bold,
To stand up and calm the pendulum sweep.
The balance is something we must try to keep.

Observe, in your care, the one who is stuck
Far in the polarity and down on their luck.
For wherever you find the extreme of a view,
The opposite is lurking not far away too.
The aim is to bring the two poles to meet.
To light up the darkness and reduce the heat.

To soften the Earth and reduce the flood.
Restoring the balance in human blood.

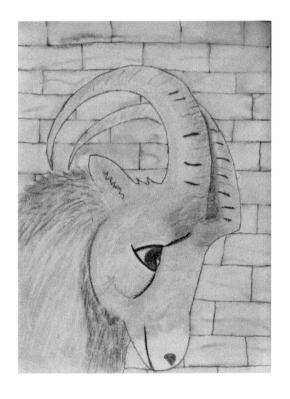

The Brick Wall

The Ram sits up.
He's hit his head.
His brow is hot,
His face is red.
His horns are ringing in his ears.
His neck displaced as well; he fears.
The wall looms tall.
The bricks are solid.
The mortar mix is also horrid.
But never fear, and don't you worry:
The Ram will work with such a hurry.
Springs to his feet,
He gives a sniff,
I'll have wall down in just a jiff.
A longer path is all I need
To take a run at greater speed.
He paces back along the path,
Stamps his feet and gives a laugh.
He takes the run and hits the wall,
That continues looming large and tall.
It throws dear Ram into backward flight.
The land looms large within his sight.
He hits the ground with such a bump,
His forehead forms a hardened lump.

The wall's too strong for this run-in.
The Ram must see he cannot win.
It's time to take a different view.
Preserve the self – so very true.
Look at the wall a different way.
A problem that won't go away
Can provide a project,
A challenge too,
Creating something completely new.

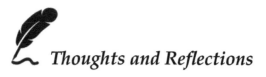 *Thoughts and Reflections*

Passing Over

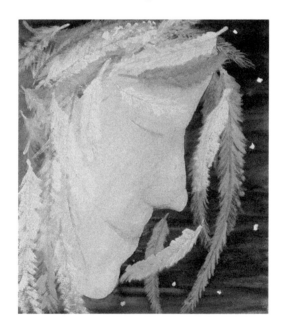

We will all face death when it is our time. We don't have much say in the matter. Believing there is something to move on to is fundamental to some. To others it is a ludicrous notion. Believing, whether it is true or not, gives us hope. Whether it is true or not is irrelevant to feeling at peace in faith.

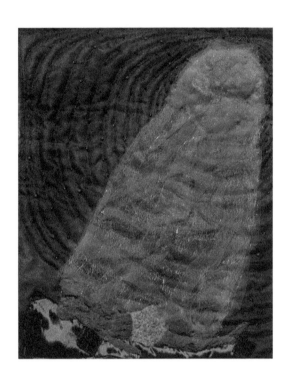

Lifting the veil

Lie quietly on your pillow.
Breathe calmly.
Breathe gently.
Be at ease in the peace.
Relax your muscles.
Let all tension go.
Let it go!
Let it go.

Do not fear.
You are not alone.
We are with you unconditionally until the time is right.
Be proud of all you have achieved.
Have no regrets, for everything has a purpose and takes its
course.
Know that you are loved so very much.
Know that your loved ones will be supported and directed
according to God's will.

Feel your body on the bed.
Know that your body is a house,
A temporary house for your spirit.
Know that your spirit will leave this house at the right time.
Don't fret.

Don't resist.
Just be.

Picture the veil.
So bright. So ethereal. So fine.
So beautiful.
The divide so comforting.
The way home.
They are there for you,
Just there, just beyond the veil.
They are there.
They promised to be there.
They are waiting for you.
They will move with you.
Go freely.
Don't resist.
Go peacefully.
Don't challenge.
Go bravely, go surely, go smoothly.
Accept.
Glide over so wonderfully.
You will be free of suffering.
At one. In bliss.

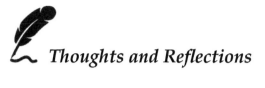

Thoughts and Reflections

Chakra

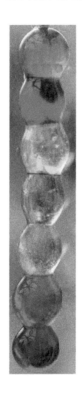

Chakra are believed to be our energy centres. They form part of the non-physical body, according to a belief that originated in the Hindu religion some centuries ago. They are considered to be important in yoga and meditation. In modern Mind Body Spirit teachings, each of the seven chakra corresponds to one of the seven colours of the rainbow and a level of consciousness. In the poems that follow, I have tried to show the key points associated with each.

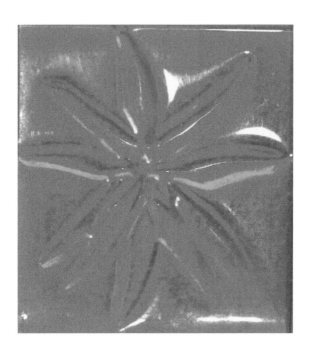

Red Chakra

Tormented, ousted, unstable.
Thrown out in the world.
Unable to stand, to defend.
The world upended.
It's shocking, traumatic; humiliated,
Defriended.
Esteem all-time low,
Pride relinquished.
Assets, property, frozen.
Extinguished.

No longer sheltered –
By the group or the tribe.
Position lost, needing to hide.
Worldly riches dwindle away.
Kudos, status, no longer an issue.
Dish of the day?
Tears with a tissue.

Physical injury, shocking event.
Haemorrhage, torture?
Some may repent.
Others take joy in the cruel blow
To destroy another,
To violently overthrow.

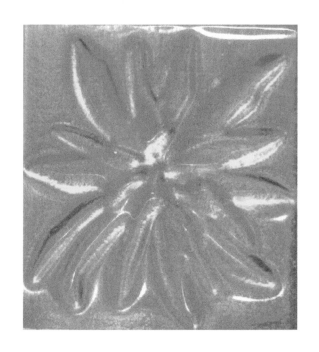

Orange Chakra

Ejaculation, conception, gestation, birth.
A creative process requiring a partnership.
A courtship. Sap flowing high.
The mating season.
A reason to conjugate, procreate.

Projects housing part of our soul,
We steer them and fill them with love, with pride.
Ambition results in fruition. Euphoria and ecstasy.
Gametes fuse! The seeds are planted.
We'll reap the harvest, which glows in orange light.
Everything's alright until it's not.

No gain equals pain, defeat and shame.
It didn't work out. Wracked with guilt.
Projects slip away like water-laden silt.
Thus is the human need to breed,
To succeed and to bathe in
The glory of the orange light.

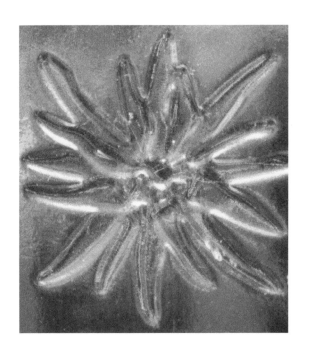

Yellow Chakra

Closely guarded inner self
Sits doggedly therein
Amongst the liver, pancreas,
Gall bladder. There's no win.
There is a constant tussle.
Over, Under, what's the mood?
Over sits in anger, self-assertive,
And quite rude.
Under lacks resilience
To stand on own two feet.
They'll need the help of others
To walk along the street.
Self-esteem is lacking.
Self-respect at an all-time low.
They'll need approval from others
To get out of this woe.
The Inner Self must make a pact
With Over and with Under.
They need to work together,
Not stand apart, asunder.
The trick is using all the strengths
Under, Over have to give
To pull each other into balance,
Then in harmony they can live.

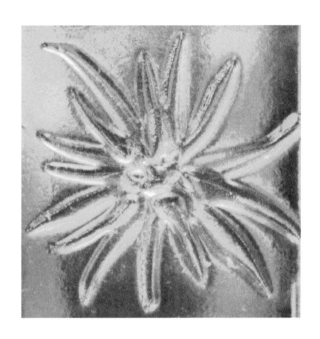

Green Chakra

Subservience to God is the right path. For he knows the plan. Surrendering your will, your plan, your ideal is a risky business but sometimes the only way. For the tide is too strong and it is wise to swim with the flow. Avoid the battle. Be kind to yourself. Love and enter the spirit of what is and not what should be because what should be is what is.

The green is the balance that love brings. Along with the heady scent of the red rose. The cross denotes the bridge between the physical and the spiritual. The crossroads between the two that reminds us we have a foot in both camps. We are spirit inhabiting a physical body.

The beating heart reflects the tussle of imbalance. Surrendering to Divine will calms the rhythm. The green can shine through brightly, calmly, lovingly. Hate has moved off and is nowhere in sight.

At ease. Free of disease.

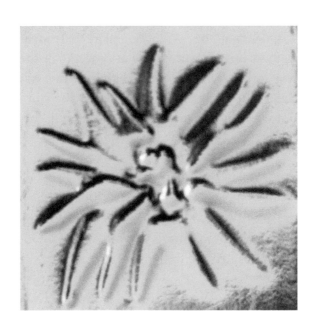

Blue Chakra

There she sits in fear and dread.
A subtle nuance, a nod of the head.
Others may sit and wonder why
The conversation has run dry.
The Truth is deep down in her throat.
She knows it very well by rote.
That demon Truth can hurt and shock;
Its strong vibrations move through rock.

But there it sits, and safely stashed,
To avoid the eventual backlash.
She squirms and wriggles to keep it in,
To camouflage and to fit in.
But festering! It can cause alarm,
Releasing local toxic harm.
She needs to reason with the brain
To restore her vocal health again.

For fitting in is not a reason;
To deny the Truth is human treason.
The brain is known to rationalise,
To delicately sympathise.
But ultimately it will form a spout
To force the hidden Truth right out.

The throat can gag, can cough, can splutter,
But soon the truth the tongue will utter.

And there it is! Relaxed and free.
At ease again for you to see.

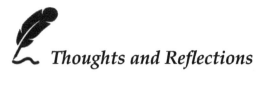 *Thoughts and Reflections*

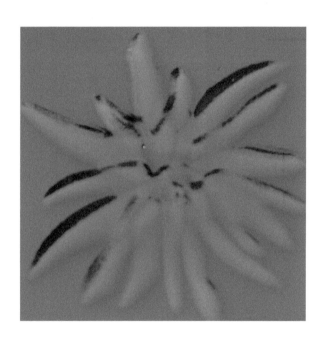

Third Eye

Seeing the indigo
Seeing the light
Seeing the truth
Blaze through night
Can't pull the wool over this eye.
Truth will be seen,
Hell 'n' heaven high.
Remote viewing may be possible here.
Flying high with the kite,
The image draws near.
Pituitary stimulated governing all.
Visions flash forward from Nice to Nepal.
Sights oh so fantastical fly magically through.
They conjure up insight and give you a view
Of past and the present and what just might be,
Of spirit and family, of you and of me!

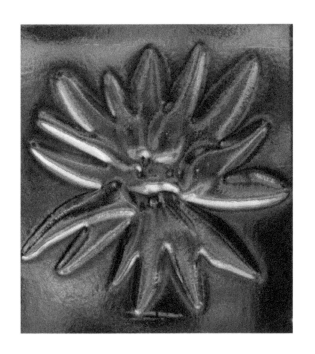

The Crown

Profoundly beautiful door of splendour,
Centred in the thousand-petal lotus,
So beautifully delicate and so tender.
Moves to open at the proper time,
Providing a bridge
From earth to divine.
Connection clear and unimpeded.
The pathway for spirit
To move when needed.
Through the violet flame they come.
A one-way path,
Opening can't be undone.
Ensure you ground
With both your feet.
Be certain
That you want to meet
The spirit guides that wait for you
To guide you
And to pull you through.

Nature

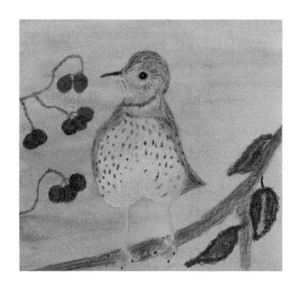

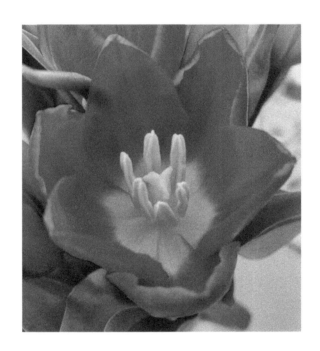

Spring Meditation

Be still. Be quiet. Be calm.
Breathe deeply.
Understand it is all planned out.
It cannot be changed. That is the way.
Leave yourself time to breathe.
And really breathe.
Do not just catch your breath.

Take time to look at the birds.
They are angelic peace bringers.
Listen to their song. Listen to the notes.
Listen to the melody.
Consider their message.
Drink the tea. But taste the tea!
Feel the ground beneath your feet.
Feel the stabilising force.
And breathe.
Hold your head high and breathe.

Look out at what is.
Be grateful for what is and breathe.
Study the flowers. The colour and the shape.
See how their movements are orchestrated in waves.
Breathe. Really breathe.

Breathe in the scent of the blossom.
The delicate perfume from flowers so pink.
Or red. Or white. So beautiful, like confetti,
That drifts into sight.
Breathe. Really breathe.

For each breath know that the beauty from without
Becomes the beauty within.
Be still and breathe. Really breathe.

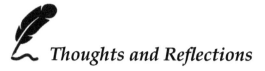

Thoughts and Reflections

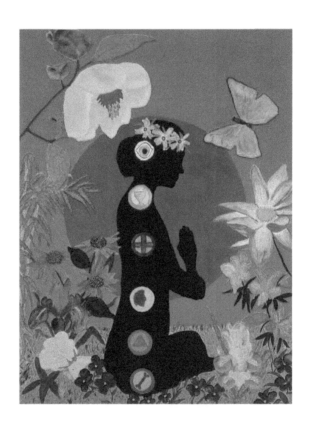

Summer Meditation

Come sit a while in this garden of mine
Where the dragonflies dart and skit in the vine.
Picture yourself with giant tree roots
That hug Mother Earth, protecting the fruits
Of their labour on high that reach to the sky
To touch wispy clouds as they pass by and by.

Visualise the red of a composite flower
That dances and prances in global wind power.
Harness the energy of the scarlet glow
To give you stability and room to grow.

There in a pot stands 'Tiger Lily'.
Her petals are orange and spotted and pretty.
Like the sun it shines out on your peaceful face
To remind you the importance of human embrace.
To touch one another, to feel the skin,
Euphoric delight, it is something akin.
Relationships, lust, safe human trust –
Creation is something we definitely must
Buy into, in some way, to fulfil our dreams.
Achievements are important, or so it seems.

Bamboo sits strongly, thick and tall,

It creates in the garden a natural wall.
View the bamboo as a supportive friend,
To carry you forward, to help you defend
The decisions you make along your path,
Avoiding, withstanding all aftermath.

Picture the delicate bud of the rose;
Imagine the bloom it's about to disclose.
The bloom is a symbol of pure love
That is felt here on Earth and high up above.
Meditate on the love you have locked in your heart;
Hold the lock in your fingers and prize it apart.
Releasing the love will make you feel better;
Send it out in the world by email or letter.

View under the tree a brilliant blue splash
Of bluebells with truth in their necks safely stashed.
Their trumpets deliver their news clear and strong,
But others might think that sometimes it's wrong.
Your energy clears like a blue summer day;
You'll feel lighter and fitter and freer this way.
There is the iris of deepest blue.
Picture it opens the third eye for you.
For here you will see truth without derision,
A series of images and strong visions.
The third eye will let you leap up and take flight,

Soar upwards on thermals as high as a kite.

In the pond floats the lotus with one thousand petals;
See this open and stabilise your very mettle.
For here your connections with spirit will fuse;
As they come close beside you, there is nothing to lose.
And here you can sit with the sun on your back.
It's warm, you are safe. There is nothing you lack.

And when you are ready to return to the now,
Become conscious of sounds that surround you somehow.
Close each flower up and give thanks to green flora.
Take a breath and realise that you've strengthened your
aura.
Open your eyes, bring yourself back into the room,
Rejuvenated, refreshed. Your life can resume.

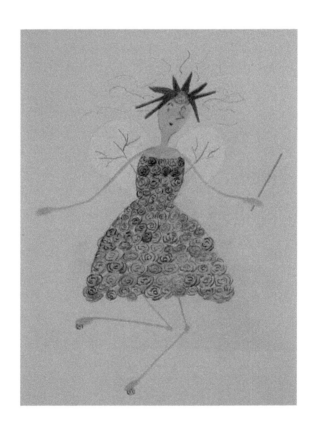

Flower Fairies

The essence of a flower is not its whorl of petals.
It's not the brewing bud encased within a round of sepals.
It's not the luscious lavender or the dusky blue.
It's not the nodding head that's been weighted by the dew.
Neither do the stamens on their own explain the fact
That the flower can calm emotions like a super magic act.
With water, energies are released by sun solarisation
To pull emotions back from extreme polarisation.
That fairy essence, with its wand, can inspire, drive and
calm
To bring you into balance, to see off any harm.
Thanks go to Dr Edward Bach for working with these
flowers,
For using fairy deep blue light to reveal their hidden
powers.
They are added to our toolbox to calm a distressed friend,
To help them with their healing, to get them on the mend.

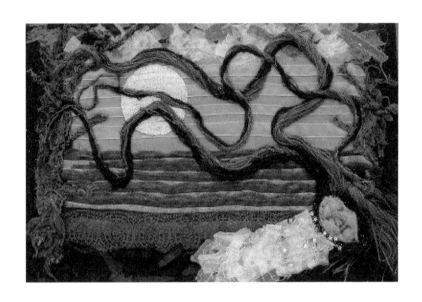

Tree Spirits

Seek refuge in the tree,
No matter what its size.
It's inhabited by spirit
To educate and guide.
Gnarly roots anchor, drawing nourishment within.
Lichen-ladened textured bark holds the nutrients in.
Twisted, bucking tree roots create a worthy seat
For man to sit and stop awhile, his sandwiches to eat.
Gaze up through the canopy, a beautiful emerald green,
Air breezing through the leaflets, meditative and serene.
Unfold the story in the dappled light.
Deliver your worry. Reveal your plight.
Tree spirits know what message to give,
Relaxing the aching heart, giving freedom to live.
Calming the nerves using source energy above,
Delivering peace, hope and love.

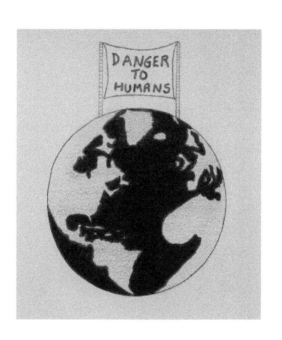

A Letter from Gaia

My spirit writes this missive by direct communication.
Do you know the depth of feeling of my complete
humiliation?
My balance is off kilter.
My rivers teem with blood.
My lungs are choked with carbon,
Biomes at risk of flood.
Thermoregulation is off set, with ice cap fridges melting.
Deserts are furnace-like and ripe for metal smelting.
My symbiotic wildlife are my living, breathing teeth.
They are hunted down for products, causing all severest
grief.
My trees that pin my skin in place are shamelessly
beheaded.
My dermis crawls and cracks and buckles. This is
something I have dreaded.
My aura has a tear above the Northern Pole.
It lets the UV rays in, a malignant growth death toll.
And what about the rubbish that restricts and chokes and
harms?
Is it not a sufficient warning or a suitable alarm?
A beautiful planet such as this,
A living breathing force
To nurture life, its purpose, is moving rapidly off course.

The human is the cause within,
A torture so intense!
He's shaved my head and burnt my skin, stuck needles in
my eyes.
He's removed my nails and spliced my guts,
Yet, I always rise.
For life on Earth is precious,
Precariously entwined.
I will preserve the order for myself but not mankind.
Homeostasis works to balance an existing fault.
As the human is the problem, I'll remove it with a jolt.

Time

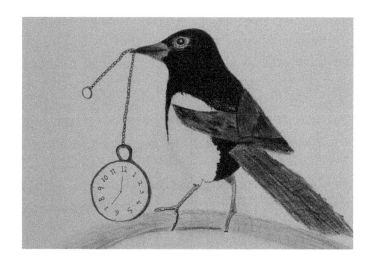

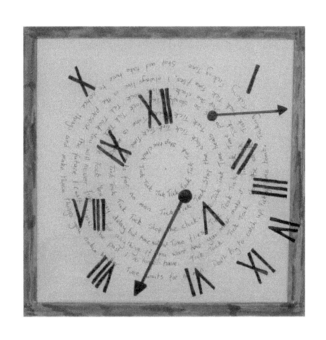

Ambiguity of Time

Tick tock, tick tock,
Stop the clock.
Tick tock, tick tock,
Stop the clock.
Hiatus.
A moment without time.
Neither forward,
Nor back.
But now.
In the present. Wrapped up with a bow.
Free from past worries,
Free from old woes.
Time gets into our heads
And under our skin.
Moves along quickly.
Doesn't know where to begin.
Time is the master, conjuring up the illusion.
Without minutes or seconds, we live in confusion.
Stop.
Take a sojourn with me!
A weightless flight
Into blue yonder without care or fear
Of missing the deadlines life puts in our way.
Without worries of where we are in the day.

Time is a permanence we wear round our necks.
Time is a moment we might choose to forget.
Time is a moment we may cherish together.
Time is ambiguous.
Time is forever!

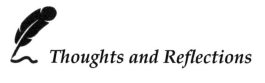 *Thoughts and Reflections*

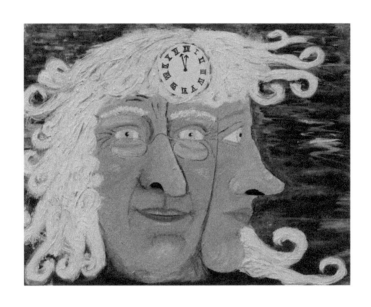

Janus

The twelfth chime beckons Janus to being,
Opening the door to the future unseeing.
Closing the door to the past good and tight,
Wishing us all a good year, a good night.

Janus blows in with gusto, his hair white and unstyled.
Two faces with eyes both excited and wild.
He carries the keys to transitioning gates;
He springs the locks then sits back and waits.

He's witnessed the past, what went wrong, what went well.
He knows there've been moments of torment, of hell!
He knows what is done can't be undone, you see.
Sometimes we have to let some things just be.

So what is the point when things have gone wrong?
When we feel we don't fit, we no longer belong.
We learn from the crisis laid bare in our hearts,
And roll out the lesson to aid future paths.

We must hope that the New Year will bring in good things:
Fortune, love and happiness to make our hearts sing.
Patience, resilience and strength when that's not enough
To help us endure when the going gets tough!

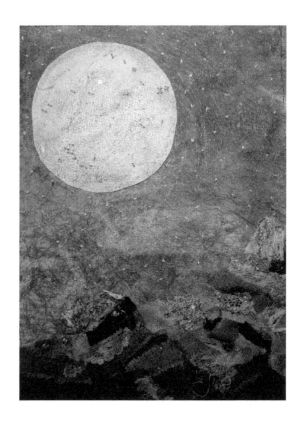

The Moon

Clothed in black sky,
Invisible and silent,
It begins its waxing journey.
The cloak slips a little to reveal
The sharpest, brightest crescent
Twinkling upon the slightest breath.
Shimmering through the grey,
It makes its way across the night.
Time and again it reappears, a little fatter,
Until its pregnant plumpness, so undeniable,
Illuminates far and wide,
Pulling the wolf, the owl, the tide.
The glow so many different shades,
A glimpse from time to time
If we are lucky.
We see myriads of moon colours,
From copper through to strawberry.
The mystical fullness is a powerful force
To cleanse the crystal,
To send out positive thoughts,
To write the cheques of universal promise,
To receive God's goodness in the gardens of biodynamic
delight.
The man in the moon

Looks on in glee
As lovers walk hand in hand quite freely
By the light that shines so brightly.
The powerful moon that guides
The ship, the whale, the shoal
Is a perfect draw for man in his rocket.
The race, to inhabit space.
But hey,
There are footprints on the surface,
And rubbish, so I am told.
With a lake without water.
Play on, fiddler.
We'll do what we ought to
And watch from afar
This beautiful feature of the night sky.
Hoorah!

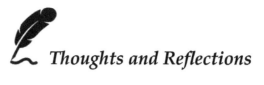 *Thoughts and Reflections*

Mystical

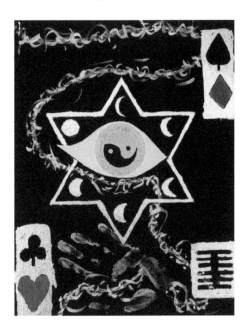

This section is for the unexplained. 'The Angel' is a real-life experience. My Grandma really was a psychic. 'I am Spirit' was channelled with eyes closed at the beginning. It was finished with eyes open. Esoteric teachings are included in this section. It emphasises the importance of sitting in the quiet to really hear spirit. The power of our thoughts is touched upon in 'Manifestation'.

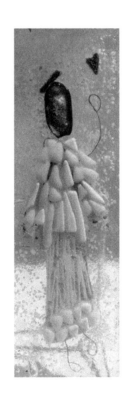

February 2021 – The Angel

And there she stood! The Angel.
In a simple lilac haze.
Her stillness reassuring,
In a near impossible phase.

Her presence so consistent,
Without obvious wing or feather.
Her form, she looked so streamlined,
It made me wonder whether
she was truly there…

But the love and comfort emanated
In a way supremely strong.
It gave me reassurance
That my thoughts could not be wrong.

'Have faith. Have love. We're here for you,'
Came the message from the being.
'We know well what you are going through.
We are powerful. We're all-seeing.'

She stayed with me the morning.
Then I left to go to work.
Apparent on the dashboard

Appeared something of a quirk.

The calendar had suffered a timely reset back:
Through the months and years and seasons,
The retreating figures
Found a knack!

For there in utmost clarity,
Gleaming green in digital fun,
Was the date the 12th of January,
Two thousand eleven, not twenty-one.

The two events together
Give me comforting proof
That the angels are close by humans,
Delivering their truth.

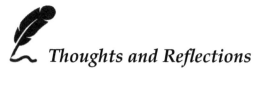 *Thoughts and Reflections*

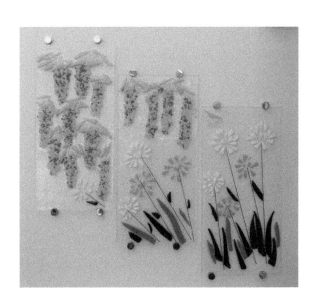

Enjoying the quiet

Steal the quiet and hold it within. Use it as a friend to hear the spirit world. They will come to you as you really listen. Do not fear. They seek out the man who sits and truly listens. Patience is required, but they will come. As sure as day follows night. Silence is your friend.

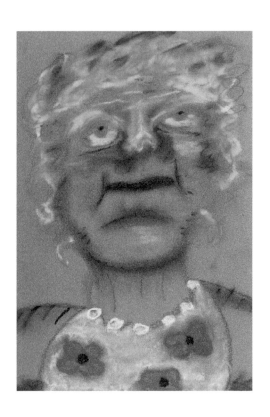

I am Spirit

In the annals of time
We move to and fro.
Unimpeded vibrational frequency.
Go!

It is time.

To experience physicality on earth.
To smell, to see.
To touch, to feel.
To speak, to hear.
To work and to love.

Learning helps us to evolve.

I am spirit on Earth,
Enjoying God's plan.
I am spirit on Earth,
Encased in the man.

And then when the journey comes to an end,

I return to spirit with a story to tell.
To reflect, to consider,

In heaven, not hell.
How to be better,
How to embrace
My failings as one of the human race.

For none of us is perfect,
And that is the point.
We develop, you see,
In our journey above.
Our ending: the frequency
Of Pure Love.

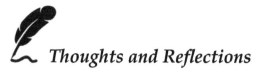 *Thoughts and Reflections*

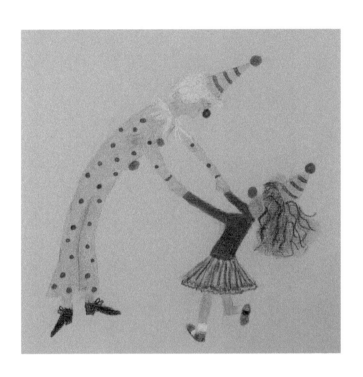

My Grandma is a Psychic

My Grandma has the whitest hair,
As pure as driven snow.
She is the kindest Grandma
That you would ever know.

She doesn't have red lips or nails,
Or a black cat, come to think.
She does have a beautiful smile, though,
And her cheeks are rosy pink.

Her kitchen smells of pastry,
The sweet and savoury kind.
She teaches me to make it short
And then to bake it blind.

And afterwards we'll sweep the floor
With an old-fashioned soft push broom.
She does not have a besom
Or a witch's black costume.

My Grandma has such fun ideas.
She plays down on the ground.
She gaily sings and dances,
And she swings me round and round.

She loves to go on outings
On the bus down into town.
She loves to play at dressing up
As a fairy or a clown.

My Grandma has a special trait,
She has the gift of sight.
She can see the mist of spirit,
And she can talk with them all night.

This gift came on her birthday
When she was just a girl.
She would sit and talk to angels,
Who'd appear in golden swirl.

My Grandma is a psychic,
She has a crystal ball.
It sits upon a wooden box
On a stand, out in the hall.

It sparkles and it glistens
As she takes a peek within.
It builds into a picture,
And a reading does begin.

My Grandma is a kindly soul,
She does not mean to fright.
Her wish to help is all she asks,
And she wishes with all her might.

She reads the playing cards for folk
Who queue right down the path.
She tells them things that make them cry
But also make them laugh!

I think I'm like my Grandma,
I see people in the room.
I can taste their favourite dinner.
I can smell their sweet perfume.

I can hear their soft, soft message
As it moves around my ear.
They have a good intention,
And so I have no fear.

Grandma says it's only spirit,
An angel come to call.
And when I get a little older
I will have her crystal ball.

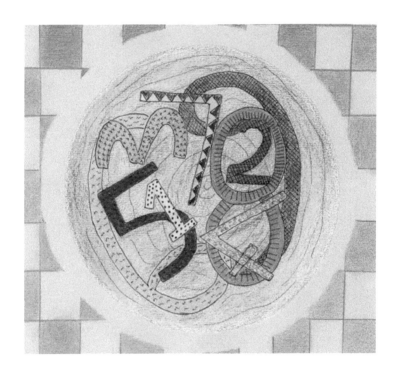

Numerology Soup

Desire carries Zero through the numerology soup.
It has a vacant centre and an edge that loops the loop.
It holds the key to newness, a wish that you can set.
All help is in close range for you to make those goals be
met.
The circle indicates an ending that will be
Quickly followed by a beginning for one and all to see.

First Number One so tall and straight,
First in the line and first at the gate.
New ventures beckon, new ideas.
Foremost direction; lastly fears.
Your confidence beams like a bolt of streak lightning,
Your projects successful and so exciting.

Gliding in Number Two with a different feeling.
Dependence on another is their way of being.
The image of a swan can be traced in their shape.
Swans pair for life; it's a hard bond to break.
A partnership, coupling, union – call it what you must –
Is suggested in the cards, a strong partnership to trust.

Trinity beckons the Number Three.
Father, Son and Holy Ghost is key.

You are urged to stay alert when spirit comes calling.
They are bringing God's message or vital warning.
Stand clear in your mind; you have been well selected
To deliver the message purely, unaffected.

Maturity accompanies the Number Four.
Picture a table on an oak floor.
Stability reigns as it should,
With each of the legs gripped tight to the wood.
Here we can sit on round-back chairs,
Discussing an issue without grace or airs.
Constancy, firmness, bring heart-ease
To a time in our lives when we strive for Peace.

Number Five tiptoes forth in an uncertain way.
One foot is with spirit, one foot in the clay.
The land it is shifting. 'Unpredictable sod!'
It brings home the truth, the certainty in God.
Be wary of life's secrets, Pentagonal One.
Strengthen links with spirit.
These can't be undone.

Responsible Six appears to push through,
Secures foundations with mortar and glue.
Sensitivity, gratitude, a generous being,
Will send greed, sloth and selfishness out the door fleeing.

Their aim is to make a home that's steadfast,
With high levels of integrity that are born to last.

Seven arrives in spiritual splendour,
Spiritual gifts overflowing. Remember
Life path is clear. Deep purpose, crystalline
Manifestation auspicious, in tune with the Divine.
Thoughts closely guarded to a positive spin,
There's not a lot that Number Seven can't win.

Prosperous Eight bounds forth, holding the purse.
They know that the issue no longer gets worse.
Job applications fly to success.
Stocks, bonds and shares soar, reducing the stress.
Number Eight is the number of balance and steadiness.
Plump, round and joyful! Now wait in readiness.

Single Number Nine, vibration all-time high,
Comes through with the Trinity from God's house in the
sky.
It reminds you there's a purpose to the path that you must
tread.
It's time to sit and listen to what is being said.
It's time to take the action to realise life's aim,
Time to work with spirit to restore Earth's love again.

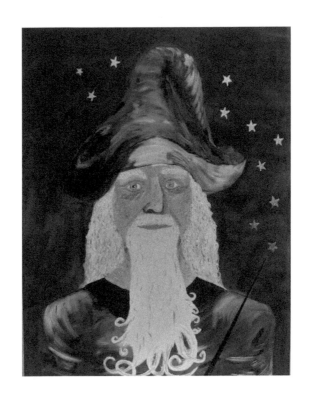

Manifestation

Merlin cloaked in purple,
As silver stars abound,
Has a wizard's wand and sceptre
And a cauldron big and round.

He has unearthly powers
That may involve his rings.
He's a prophet! He's a bard!
He's advisor to the Kings.

A Welshman good and proper,
Seeing dragons in the air.
He works as God's servant,
Playing hard but playing fair.

He is innately human.
They say his mother was a nun.
But legend of his Father
Would make some want to run.

But keep that in perspective.
He is the archetype
Where good will overthrow evil
When the time is good and ripe.

He is the natural healer,
The 'Shaman in the Wood'.
A working Priest of Nature,
Using herbs just as he should.

He did succumb to passion
For the 'Lady in the Lake',
But unrequited love
Merlin's faculties did take.

It left the wizard powerless
In the heart of forest thick.
He could not move his being
Through to health from deeply sick.

We are left with Merlin's legend
And his healing legacy.
We can visualise his power
To move a project from A to B.

His goodness can flow through us,
Stoking up our glowing fires.
It can help us raise our energy,
Manifesting our desires

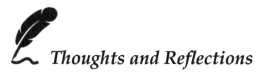 *Thoughts and Reflections*

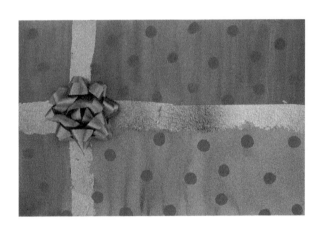

About the Author

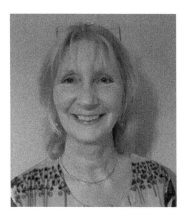

Karen Old

Growing up with my grandmother, a psychic medium, was an interesting time! We had an assortment of visitors seeking help and advice. Guidance would come from the standard playing cards, the angel board, tea leaves and the aura. Spirit would drop in from time to time to deliver reassurance. It was something I was used to and deeply respectful of.

My grandmother was the sweetest person you could ever wish to meet. She had the innate 'gift'. She could read with great accuracy, and as a young lady's maid, she was often called to read for the 'lady of the house'. Her passing was a tragic loss and I still miss her every day.

After her death, my own spiritual development was to remain dormant until much later. I had some issues to resolve and needed to connect with my deceased father. I found peace after visiting a brilliant medium, Nicola Hall, but I also began to retrieve my own psychic abilities. For several years now, I have been developing and honing my skills as a medium by attending regular training and supervision sessions.

My working life has been varied. I have worked as a nurse, teacher and homeopath.

Milton Keynes UK
Ingram Content Group UK Ltd.
UKHW051925100823
426667UK00009B/158